18 Useful Suggestions on How to Reduce fat around your midsection.

A tutorial on how to reduce fat in the abdominal region

By

Marci R. Vaughn

Disclaimer

No part of this book may be reproduced or transmitted in any form or by any means, electronic or mechanical, including photocopying, recording or by any information storage and retrieval system, without written permission from the author."

Table of contents

Introduction

An excessive amount of abdominal fat is associated with an increased risk of developing certain chronic illnesses. You can reduce the amount of belly fat you have by, among other things, cutting back on alcohol consumption, increasing the amount of protein you eat, and lifting weights. Having much fat in the abdominal region can have a detrimental effect on health and may be a contributing factor in the development of various persistent diseases.

Visceral fat, a specific kind of abdominal fat, is a key risk factor for type 2 diabetes as well as heart disease and other illnesses. The body mass index, sometimes known as BMI, is used by a variety of health organizations to categorize weight and determine the likelihood of developing metabolic diseases. The Body Mass Index (BMI) does not take into consideration body composition or visceral fat because it is only calculated using a person's height and weight.

In spite of the fact that losing fat in this region might be challenging, there are a few different things you can try if you want to minimize the amount of abdominal fat you have. This article discusses the reasons for having belly fat, the issues that come along with it, and some effective strategies for losing belly fat.

Part I

What exactly is meant by the term "belly fat"?

The term "belly fat" refers to the fat that collects around the abdomen. There are two different kinds of abdominal fat:

- Visceral fat is the type of fat that surrounds an individual's organs.
- Subcutaneous fat is fat that is located just under the surface of the skin.

In most cases, the health risks associated with visceral fat are significantly higher than those associated with having subcutaneous fat. Alterations to one's way of life, on the other hand, can frequently assist individuals in lowering their abdominal fat levels and improving their general   health.

Part II

What can cause belly Fat?

People put on belly fat for a variety of reasons, the most common of which are bad dietary habits, insufficient physical activity, and emotional stress. People can lose belly fat by making adjustments to their lifestyle, such as improving their eating, being more active, and making other changes.

Unhealthy diet

When a person consumes more calories than they burn off over a prolonged period of time, this can lead to weight gain as well as an increase in the amount of fat that is stored in the body.

Because of this, diets that are high in calories but low in nutrients might increase the likelihood that a person will put on extra weight and have a higher percentage of abdominal fat.

As a result of the fact that fats contain the maximum number of calories per gram, eating fats might speed up the rate at which a person consumes additional calories. Foods that are high in sugar and processed foods are major contributors to weight gain and obesity. These types of foods can also slow a person's metabolism, which can make it more difficult to lose fat.

A lack of physical activity (exercise) The amount of physical activity a person does is the second-most important factor in the energy in versus energy out equation.

The biggest contributor to both obesity and an increase in the percentage of body fat that one carries is a lack of physical exercise. Putting on extra weight and leading a sedentary lifestyle both make it more difficult for a person to begin an exercise routine.

If a person consumes more calories than they burn off through physical activity, then their body will store the excess calories as fat.

Excessive amounts of alcohol
Drinking an excessive amount of alcohol can lead to a variety of health issues, including liver illness and inflammation.

Regardless of a person's body mass index (BMI) or other markers, higher levels of alcohol use have been associated with higher levels of visceral fat, according to research that was conducted on the relationship between obesity and alcohol consumption. The researchers discovered no discernible connection between drinking alcohol and having a higher percentage of subcutaneous fat.

The   Strain
The steroid hormone known as cortisol assists the body in managing stress and keeping it under control. A person's

metabolism can be affected by the hormone cortisol, which is released by the body whenever they are in a stressful or potentially harmful scenario.

When people are feeling worried, they frequently seek solace in the form of food. Because of cortisol, the body stores those extra calories around the abdomen and in other parts of the body for use at a later time.

What is Genetics?
There is some evidence to suggest that a person's genetic makeup can influence whether or not they will develop obesity. According to a reputable source, scientists believe that genes can have an effect on behavior, metabolism, and the chance of acquiring obesity-related disorders.

A person's probability of getting fat is also influenced by both their conduct and their surrounding environment.

Inadequate **Sleep**

According to the findings of certain studies, a decrease in the typical amount of time spent sleeping is associated with an increase in visceral body fat.

A decrease in the amount of time spent sleeping is associated with an increase in the amount of food consumed, which may contribute to the accumulation of fat in the abdomen region.

The inability to get sufficient quality sleep can also contribute to poor eating practices, such as emotional eating, which can have negative consequences.

Part III

Why Should You Be Afraid of Belly Fat?

One of the primary factors contributing to the development of major diseases is obesity (belly fat). The presence of excess abdominal fat has been linked to an increased risk of:

- coronary artery disease
- attacks on the heart
- hypertension; high blood pressure
- the stroke
- Diabetes type 2 (T2D)
- allergic rhinitis
- cancer of the breast
- carcinoma of the colon
- Alzheimer's disease

Part IV

Tips That Actually Work To Reduce Belly Fat

Here is a list of 18 things to perform in order to reduce abdominal fat:

1. **Consume a diet rich in soluble fiber.** When combined with water, soluble fiber produces a gel that acts as a barrier to prevent the rapid movement of food through the digestive tract.

According to studies, this fiber may help you lose weight by making you feel full for longer, which in turn leads to you eating less naturally. Insoluble fiber, on the other hand, may assist in the reduction of belly fat. An older observational study that involved over 1,100 adults indicated that for every 10-gram (g) increase in soluble fiber intake, belly fat accumulation decreased by 3.7% over the course of 5 years.

- fresh produce
- fruits and veggies
- Legume crops
- oats
- malted barley

By making you feel fuller for longer and preventing the absorption of additional calories, soluble fiber may facilitate weight loss. Your diet should focus on including plenty of foods that are high in fiber.

2. Steer clear of meals that are high in trans fats.
In order to produce trans fats, hydrogen is injected into unsaturated fats like soybean oil. Examples of these fats are palm oil and peanut oil. Previously, they might have been discovered in certain margarines and spreads, and they were also frequently added to packaged goods. However, the majority of food manufacturers have discontinued using them in their products.

In observational and experimental research, these lipids have been shown to be associated with inflammation, heart disease, insulin resistance, and the accumulation of belly fat.

3. **Drink alcohol in moderation for optimal health.**

A moderate quantity of alcohol consumption may be beneficial to one's health, but drinking too much alcohol may be detrimental to one's health. According to the findings of several studies, drinking too much alcohol may contribute to belly obesity.

Studies that use observations as their method of data collection relate heavy alcohol use to a greatly increased likelihood of acquiring extra fat accumulation around the waist. Cutting back on alcohol consumption can perhaps assist in reducing your waist size. You don't have to give it up entirely, but cutting back on the total amount you consume in a single day can be helpful.

In one investigation into the effects of alcohol consumption, over 2,000 participants took part. Those who drank alcohol on a daily basis but had an average of fewer than one drink of alcohol per day had less belly fat compared to those who drank less frequently but consumed more alcohol on the days that they did drink. It is advised that males restrict their daily alcohol consumption to no more than two drinks and that women limit their consumption to no more than one drink, as stated in the most recent version of the Dietary Guidelines for Americans.

There is a correlation between drinking too much alcohol and having a larger waist circumference. If you are aiming to reduce your body fat percentage, you should either drink alcohol in moderation or altogether abstain from it.

4. **Consume a diet that is rich in protein.**
When it comes to maintaining a healthy
weight, protein is a component that cannot
be overlooked. Consuming a lot of protein
triggers a greater release of the hormone
peptide YY, which in turn reduces the
amount of food that one wants to eat and
makes one feel more full.

Protein not only speeds up your
metabolism but also assists in the
maintenance of your muscle mass, even as
you reduce your overall body fat
percentage. Numerous observational
studies have found that individuals who
consume a diet high in protein have a
reduced prevalence of belly fat compared
to those who consume a diet low in
protein. Make sure that each meal has a
good supply of protein, like one of the
following: meat, fish, eggs, dairy
products., protein extracted from whey,
faba beans.

If you're attempting to reduce the amount of fat that you carry around your middle, eating meals that are high in protein but not too fatty, like fish, lean meat, and beans, could be effective.

5. **Reduce the amount of stress in your life.**

Because it stimulates the adrenal glands to create cortisol, often known as the stress hormone, stress might cause you to gain weight around the abdominal area. According to research, elevated levels of cortisol both stimulate appetite and promote the storage of belly fat.

In addition, women who already have a large waist have a tendency to create more cortisol in reaction to stress than women who do not have a large waist. An increase in cortisol is another factor that contributes to an increase in abdominal fat. Participating in stress-relieving activities can assist in the reduction of belly fat.

Yoga and meditation both have the potential to be helpful practices.

6. Eat fewer foods that are high in sugar.

When ingested in excessive amounts, fructose is associated with a number of chronic diseases and sugar may include this substance.

These conditions include cardiovascular disease, diabetes type 2, and nonalcoholic fatty liver disease. It is essential to understand that consumption of refined sugar is not the only factor that can contribute to an increase in abdominal fat. Even sweeteners that come from natural sources, such as honey made from actual flowers, should be consumed in moderation.

A significant number of people put on excess weight because they consume an excessive amount of sugar. Reduce the amount of candy and processed meals you eat because they contain a lot of added sugar.

7. Perform some form of aerobic activity (cardio).
Aerobic exercise, also known as "cardio," is an excellent approach to both enhancing one's health and reducing one's caloric intake. The abdominal fat can be effectively reduced by using cardio as a form of exercise. On the other hand, the findings are inconclusive on which level of physical activity is more beneficial: moderate or high intensity. In any event, the duration and frequency of your workout routine are both potential factors that can have a significant impact.

According to the findings of one study, postmenopausal women who participated in aerobic activity for 300 minutes per week shed more fat from all areas of their bodies compared to those who only exercised for 150 minutes per week. Researchers did notice, however, that changes in visceral abdominal fat were not statistically different between the two groups.

8. **Reduce your consumption of carbohydrates, particularly refined carbs.**

If you want to lose fat, including abdominal fat, cutting back on the amount of carbohydrates you eat can be quite helpful. Persons who are overweight, persons who are at risk for developing type 2 diabetes, and people who have polycystic ovarian syndrome (PCOS) may find that following a low-carb diet helps them lose belly fat.

You are not required to stick to a very rigorous low-carb diet. It has been shown by some bodies of research that substituting refined carbohydrates for unprocessed starchy carbohydrates may improve metabolic health and lead to a reduction in abdominal obesity. The Framingham Heart Study found that those whose diets consisted primarily of whole grains had a 17% lower risk of having excess belly fat compared to individuals whose diets consisted primarily of diets that were high in refined grains.

High consumption of refined carbohydrates has been linked to an excessive amount of abdominal fat. Think about cutting back on the amount of carbohydrates you eat or replacing the refined carbohydrates in your diet with healthier forms of carbohydrates, including whole grains, legumes, or vegetables.

9. Carry out resistance training, also known as lifting weights. The practice of resistance training, which includes weightlifting and other forms of strength training, is essential for maintaining and enhancing one's muscle mass.

According to the findings of research that included participants with prediabetes, type 2 diabetes, and fatty liver disease, resistance exercise may also be useful for the removal of abdominal fat.

In fact, research conducted on adolescents who were overweight revealed that a combination of strength training and aerobic exercise resulted in the highest reduction in visceral fat. This finding was found in the study. Should you choose to begin lifting weights, it is highly recommended that you first consult a medical professional and then seek the guidance of a licensed personal trainer.

Lifting weights is an effective method for losing weight and may be especially helpful in reducing abdominal fat. According to the findings of several studies, it is considerably more efficient when combined with aerobic activity.

10. **Reduce your consumption of beverages with added sugar.** Beverages that are sweetened with sugar have a high concentration of added sugars such as fructose, which can contribute to the accumulation of fat in the abdominal region.

When compared to ingesting less than one serving of sugar-sweetened beverages per week, participants in a study of adults with type 2 diabetes who consumed at least one portion of sugar-sweetened beverages each week had greater amounts of abdominal fat. In addition, because your brain does not absorb liquid calories in the same way that it does solid ones, you are more likely to consume an excessive amount of calories in the future, which will result in your body storing those extra calories as fat.

If you want to shed weight around your midsection, the greatest thing you can do is cut back on sugary drinks like these:

soda, hit (punch), Iced or sweetened tea, Mixers for alcoholic beverages that contain sugar.

If you want to reduce the amount of fat stored in your abdominal region, one of the most significant things you can do is cut back on liquid forms of sugar, such as sugar-sweetened beverages.

11. **Get a good night's sleep every night.** Getting enough sleep is critical for many different elements of one's health, including their weight. According to a number of studies, not getting enough sleep may be associated with an increased risk of obesity as well as an increase in abdominal fat for certain demographics.

The medical problem known as sleep apnea, in which one has brief pauses in breathing while sleeping, has also been connected to having an excessive amount of visceral fat. In addition to sleeping for at least seven hours each night, you also need to make sure that the quality of your sleep is sufficient. If you think you could have sleep apnea or another type of sleep problem, you should discuss potential treatments with your primary care physician.

There is a correlation between not getting enough sleep and an increased risk of gaining weight. If you are wanting to shed some pounds, it is imperative that you get adequate quality sleep each night.

12. **Keep a record of the food you eat and the exercise you do.** There are a lot of different things that can help you lose weight and belly fat, but the most important thing is to consume fewer calories than your body requires for weight maintenance. You can better keep track of the number of calories you consume by maintaining a food journal, utilizing an online meal tracker or app, or both.

It has been demonstrated that following this technique can aid in the process of weight loss. In addition, food monitoring tools make it easier for you to monitor your consumption of macro- and micronutrients like protein, carbohydrates, and fiber. A lot of them also let you keep track of your workouts and other kinds of physical activity. On this page, you will find links to a number of free mobile applications and websites that may be used to keep track of the calories and nutrients that you consume.

If you are trying to shed some pounds, keeping track of the food that you consume might be an effective tool. Keeping a meal journal or making use of an online food tracker are two of the most common approaches to accomplishing this goal.

13. **Eat a few servings of fatty fish per week.**

A diet that is well-balanced may benefit

from the inclusion of fatty fish as a source of nutrition. They include a lot of high-quality protein as well as omega-3 fats, both of which have been linked to a reduced risk of developing chronic diseases. There is some evidence that consuming foods rich in omega-3 fatty acids may also help reduce visceral fat.

Aim to consume between two and three portions of fatty fish every week. Some excellent options are:

- the salmon
- the herring
- the sardine
- jack mackerel
- sardines or anchovies

Supplements containing plant-based omega-3 fatty acids, produced from sources such as algae, are also available for individuals who don't routinely consume fish, as well as vegans and vegetarians.

It's possible that your overall health can be improved by eating fatty fish or taking omega-3 supplements that come from fish oil or algae. There is some indication that it may also lower the amount of belly fat that people with fatty liver disease have.

14. **Reduce the amount of fruit juice you drink.**

Despite the fact that it contains essential vitamins and minerals, fruit juice typically has a sugar content that is comparable to that of soda and other sweetened beverages. For instance, an 8-ounce serving (248 milliliters) of unsweetened apple juice has 24 grams of sugar, with fructose accounting for more than half of the total.

Fruit juice often has the same amount of sugar as soda, and as a result, excessive use of the beverage can lead to weight gain. It is in your best interest to consume a moderate amount and to also enjoy other beverages, such as water or iced tea that is unsweetened.

15. **Consume probiotic foods or take a supplement containing probiotics.** Some meals and dietary supplements include live bacteria known as probiotics. They might offer certain health benefits, such as assisting in the improvement of digestive health and boosting immune function.

Researchers have discovered that different species of bacteria each play a part in the regulation of one's weight and that maintaining the appropriate bacterial balance can aid in the process of weight loss, including the reduction of abdominal fat. Members of the Lactobacillus family, such as Lactobacillus fermentum, Lactobacillus amylovorus, have been proven to lower the amount of fat that is stored in the abdominal region.

However, despite the fact that probiotics might be helpful for weight loss, additional research is required. Before adding probiotics or any other supplements to your daily routine, it is essential to discuss your options with a medical professional. This is because the Food and Drug Administration does not regulate all probiotics.

16. **Think about doing a fast every so often.**

As a means of shedding excess pounds, intermittent fasting has recently seen a surge in popularity. It's a pattern of eating that alternates between times of eating and periods of not eating at regular intervals.

One of the more common approaches is to abstain from food for twenty-four hours once or twice every week. Another method involves abstaining from food every day for 16 hours and then consuming all of your meals in a span of 8 hours. Bear in mind that there is some data suggesting that intermittent fasting may have a negative effect on blood sugar control in women but not in men. However, men are not affected by this in the same way. Stop fasting immediately if you feel any bad consequences, even though some modified forms of intermittent fasting appear to be healthier options. In addition, you should see a medical professional before attempting intermittent fasting or making any other dietary adjustments.

A strategy of eating known as intermittent fasting involves going without food for set amounts of time at regular intervals. According to a number of studies, it may be one of the most efficient techniques to get rid of abdominal fat as well as excess weight.

17. **Consume some green tea.** Drinking green tea is one of the healthiest things you can do. Caffeine and an antioxidant known as epigallocatechin

gallate (EGCG) are both present, and both are thought to stimulate metabolic activity. EGCG is a catechin, and various studies have suggested that it may assist in the loss of abdominal fat. Consuming green tea in conjunction with physical activity may have a synergistic impact that is more pronounced.

A single study came to the intriguing conclusion that drinking green tea can hasten weight loss, particularly when it is done in amounts of less than 500 milligrams per day for a period of 12 weeks. According to the findings of another study (74), drinking green tea on a regular basis may be advantageous for reducing both total body weight and the size of the waistline. Nevertheless, there is a need for additional study of higher quality.

Even though additional research is needed, consuming green tea on a regular basis has been linked to a reduction in body fat. On its own, however, it is probably not as beneficial as when combined with physical activity, which is why it is recommended.

18. Make adjustments to your way of life and integrate a variety of approaches.

It's possible that doing only one of the tasks on this list won't have much of an impact on its own.

It's possible that combining multiple approaches will produce the best overall outcomes. It's interesting to note that many of these approaches are often related to eating in a balanced way and living a healthy lifestyle overall. Consequently, modifying your lifestyle in a way that is sustainable over the long run is an essential component of shedding your belly fat and keeping it off. The decrease in body fat is often an unintended but natural consequence of adopting more healthful behaviors, maintaining an active lifestyle, and eating less food that has been highly   processed.

Conclusion

You can get rid of abdominal fat by employing tactics such as going for a daily run that lasts for 25 minutes and eating a balanced diet. The ability of the body to burn fat more efficiently is facilitated by following a diet that is low in calories, fats, and sweets.

In addition, if you want to lose belly fat rapidly, you should undertake abdominal workouts because they will tone the abdominal muscles and improve the appearance of the abdomen.

9 798866 887859